FERTILITY DIET COOKBOOK

OVER 50 DAYS OF DELICIOUS RECIPES TO NATURALLY BOOST OVULATION AND IMPROVE CHANCES OF PREGNANCY

STEVE BELL

TABLE OF CONTENT

INTRODUCTION

Understanding Fertility

Key Nutrients for Boosting Ovulation

Meal Planning Tips

Breakfast Recipes

- Nutrient-packed Smoothie Bowls
- Energizing Breakfast Wraps
- Protein-rich Pancakes

Lunch Ideas

- Quinoa Salad with Fertility Boosting Veggies
- Grilled Chicken and Avacado Wrap
- Lentil Soup for Balanced Nutrition

Serve the lentil soup with a side of whole-grain bread for a complete and satisfying meal. Dinner Delights

- Salmon with Roasted Sweet Potatoes
- Vegetarian Stir-Fry with Tofu
- Whole Grain Pasta Primavera

Snacks

- Fertility-Boosting Trail Mix
- Greek Yogurt Parfait
- Homemade Energy Bars

Desserts with a Purpose

- Berry Bliss Smoothie Pops
- Dark Chocolate Avocado Mousse
- Fruit Salad with Mint

Lifestyle Tips for Fertility

Weekly Meal Plan
Grocery Shopping Guide
Conclusion

INTRODUCTION

Thank you for visiting the "Fertility Diet Cookbook: Over 50 Days of Delicious Recipes to Naturally Boost Ovulation and Improve Chances of Pregnancy." I'm excited to start this life-changing adventure with you, one that is based on the idea that what we eat has a significant impact on our ability to conceive.

Being the author of this cookbook, I have a personal interest in nutrition and how it affects reproductive health. My spouse and I struggled with infertility years ago. It was a road that was not without its share of emotions, uncertainty, and moments of powerlessness. Amid visits to the doctor and prescriptions, we learned about the empowering impact of a fertility-focused diet.

We investigated the complex relationship between diet and reproductive health as a result of our knowledge-seeking. We delved into the realm of healthful, nutrient-dense foods that satisfied our palates and gave our bodies the fundamental components needed for conceiving. By trial and error and a little bit of culinary ingenuity, we saw improvements in our health and, in the end, the happy news of a successful pregnancy.

This cookbook is a deeply felt compilation that grew out of that personal journey, which motivated me to tell you about the life-changing power of a diet centred on fertility. Every dish is created with the intention of becoming a part of your own story—a narrative about embracing fertility, embracing wellbeing, and relishing the rich tapestry of flavours life has to offer.

So come along on this gastronomic adventure with me, whether you're just starting out on your fertility journey, navigating the complicated routes to conception, or just looking for nourishment for your reproductive health. As you prepare meals meant to fulfil your aspirations of a happy, healthy family, use the pages of this cookbook to serve as a source of motivation, wisdom, and maybe even a hint of magic.

Cheers to your trip, which I hope is full of delicious food, good health, and the possibility of fresh starts.

Understanding Fertility

Knowledge becomes a potent ally in the complex web of fertility, shedding light on the road to pregnancy. This chapter explores the complex topic of reproductive health in further detail, providing an in-depth analysis of the variables that affect fertility as well as the critical role that diet plays in maximising your chances of becoming pregnant.

1. The Complexity of Fertility: Hormonal balance, ovulatory function, lifestyle decisions, and environmental influences are just a few of the many aspects that affect fertility, which is a complex phenomenon. This section breaks down the intricacies of fertility, offering insights into the intricate dance of hormones and the different elements that go into creating an environment conducive to conception.

2. Hormonal Harmony: The intricate interactions between hormones, which create a hormonal symphony that controls the menstrual cycle and

ovulation, are essential to fertility. To identify the fertile window and increase the likelihood of conception, one must have a thorough understanding of the hormonal ebb and flow. This section clarifies the complex hormonal dynamics, providing you with information that will serve as a guide for your reproductive journey.

3. The Effect of Nutrition on Fertility: In the story of fertility, nutrition is a major character. The significant impact of particular nutrients on reproductive health is examined in this section. Every nutrient, from antioxidants and omega-3 fatty acids to vital vitamins and minerals, has a specific function in promoting ovulation, preserving hormonal balance, and fostering an environment that is favourable to fertility.

4. Fertility-Boosting Foods: Expanding upon the basics of nutritional knowledge, this section presents a variety of foods that increase fertility. Every dietary category has been carefully chosen to improve fertility, from lean proteins that

supply amino acids to leafy greens that are high in folate. Explore the realm of vibrant veggies, complete grains, and lean meats as we unravel the nutritional composition that supports the health of your reproductive system.

5. Lifestyle Factors: In addition to diet, lifestyle decisions have a big impact on fertility. The effects of variables like stress, sleep, and exercise on reproductive health are examined in this section. Gaining knowledge about how these factors interact with fertility can help you create a comprehensive strategy that goes beyond the plate.

6. Environmental Factors: Our living conditions have a subtle influence on how fertile we become. This section examines environmental factors, such as exposure to pollutants and lifestyle choices, that may have an impact on reproductive health. Being aware of these outside factors gives you the ability to make wise decisions and creates a supportive atmosphere for conception.

7. The Fertility Emotional Landscape:
It is critical to acknowledge the subtle emotional undertones associated with conception. The psychological components of the fertility journey are examined in this part, along with the effects of stress, anxiety, and emotional wellness on reproductive health. Developing an optimistic outlook becomes essential to your all-encompassing approach to conception.

Think of this chapter as a compass that will help you navigate the treacherous landscape of fertility. Every segment serves as a springboard, providing knowledge that enables you to make decisions that are in line with your particular reproductive objectives. Gaining information about the interactions between dietary, lifestyle, and hormonal aspects sets you on a path of empowerment and gives you the ability to confidently and clearly manage the path towards conception.

Key Nutrients for Boosting Ovulation

Ovulation is a key event in the process of becoming pregnant, and it takes centre stage in the complex dance of fertility. This chapter explores the realm of nutrition, revealing the vital vitamins, minerals, and other substances that are integral to the ovulatory process and help to enhance it. Every nutrient takes centre stage in the story of fertility, from the colourful range of fruits and vegetables to the nutrient-dense assortment of proteins and fats, adding to the ovulation's melodious symphony.

1. Folate: Widely hailed as the superhero of B vitamins, folate turns out to be essential for ovulatory health. This section delves into the function of folate in promoting DNA synthesis and cell division, two critical processes that facilitate a normal ovulation cycle. Find out how much folate is in leafy greens, beans, and fortified grains, and how including these foods in your diet will help you become more fertile.

2. Omega-3 Fatty Acids: The main players in fostering hormonal balance and bolstering ovulatory function are the omega-3 fatty acids, especially EPA (eicosapentaenoic acid) and DHA (docosahexaenoic acid). This section walks you through the many foods that are high in these fatty acids, such as walnuts, flaxseeds, and fatty seafood like salmon and mackerel. As you add foods high in omega-3 fatty acids to your diet, you'll be opening up a vast array of possibilities and creating an atmosphere that will support healthy ovulation.

3. Antioxidants: Antioxidants are partners in the pursuit of a healthy ovulation because they protect the body from oxidative stress. Explore the vibrant world of fruits and vegetables, which are a great source of antioxidants such as selenium, beta-carotene, and vitamins C and E. This section explains how these substances neutralise free radicals, protecting reproductive cell integrity and increasing the chances of a successful ovulation cycle.

4. Iron: This mineral is essential for reproductive health in addition to its role in avoiding anaemia. This section delves into the role that iron plays in the transportation of oxygen, which is an essential component for the creation of energy during ovulation. Discover the various sources of iron, such as legumes, dark leafy greens, and lean meats, and discover how ovulatory energy demands are supported by optimally maintained iron levels.

5. Vitamin D: Vitamin D, the vitamin found in sunshine, comes into its own as a supporter of reproductive health and a regulator of hormonal balance. This section explains where to get vitamin D, from exposure to sunshine to fortified foods, and emphasises how crucial it is for a smooth ovulatory cycle. Examine the ways in which this vitamin contributes to the rhythm of fertility by interacting with the complex hormonal dance.

6. Zinc: In this examination of essential minerals, zinc, a trace element with significant effects on reproductive health, takes its position. Zinc is a complex participant in the ovulatory symphony, having roles in cell division, DNA synthesis, and hormone regulation. Explore the world of foods high in zinc, such as poultry, oysters, and seeds, and learn how this mineral helps to support the many processes involved in ovulation.

7. Calcium: Its importance in reproductive physiology is revealed by calcium, which goes beyond its well-known function in bone health. This section explains the role that calcium plays in muscle function, particularly in the smooth muscle contractions that occur during ovulation. Discover the calcium-rich foods and plant-based substitutes that can support your reproductive journey.

Thinking of this chapter as a nutrient-rich environment where every food category and micronutrient supports the health of your ovulatory cycle can help you navigate it. Knowing how these essential nutrients work together to boost ovulation and improve your overall reproductive health gives you the power to create a diet focused on fertility. Welcome to a gastronomic adventure where the ingredients enhance the story of your conception journey by acting as agents of fertility.

Meal Planning Tips

Starting a fertility-focused cooking journey is more than just putting ingredients together; it's a deliberate planning of meals that support your body and your reproductive goals. This chapter offers a wealth of information on meal planning, assisting you in creating menus that are harmoniously integrated into your daily routine and that are well-balanced and increasing fertility.

1. Accept Diversity and Colour: Bring life to your meals by incorporating a wide range of fruits, vegetables, whole grains, and proteins into your diet. Every hue represents a distinct combination of phytochemicals, antioxidants, and nutrients that support your general health. This tip guarantees a wide range of fertility-boosting components and improves the appearance of your meal.

2. Make Whole meals a Priority: Make whole, unprocessed meals a priority when creating your

meal plans. Lean meats like chicken, beans, and lentils, as well as nutritious grains like quinoa and brown rice, provide a nutritional powerhouse that promotes hormonal balance and reproductive health. Reduce your dependency on processed foods by using more naturally occurring ingredients.

3. Balance Macronutrients: Ensure that each meal contains a harmonious proportion of proteins, lipids, and carbohydrates. Maintaining equilibrium between these fundamental elements guarantees prolonged energy levels and establishes the basis for a comprehensive fertility diet. When planning meals, take into account lean proteins, healthy fats, and complex carbohydrates to make them filling and fulfilling.

4. Time Your Meals Wisely: Space out your meals and snacks throughout the day in a deliberate manner. To maintain steady blood sugar levels, which are essential for hormonal balance, aim for smaller, more frequent meals.

This advice promotes healthy ovulation by fostering an environment that is conducive to general wellness.

5. Hydration Matters: Water is an essential component of any diet regimen aimed at promoting fertility. Maintaining proper hydration facilitates digestion, maintains cellular activity, and facilitates the delivery of nutrients to target areas. To make sure your body functions at its best during your fertility journey, fill your day with water, herbal teas, and meals high in moisture.

6. Mindful Eating Practices: Practice mindfulness when eating by appreciating every taste and being aware of your body's signals of hunger and fullness. This technique improves your eating experience in general and helps you develop a stronger bond with the nutritious components of food. You can have a good relationship with your fertility-focused diet by practicing mindful eating.

7. Plan Ahead for Convenience: Make your travels easier by organising and cooking your meals in advance. Meal planning and batch cooking not only save time but also guarantee that fertility-boosting meals are always available, which lessens the temptation to choose less healthful options when things are hectic. Success is facilitated by having prepared ingredients in a well-stocked refrigerator.

8. Work together with foods that promote fertility:
Plan your meals to include foods that are recognised to increase fertility. Add leafy greens, seafood high in omega-3 fatty acids, and berries high in antioxidants to your weekly diet. With the help of this suggestion, meal planning becomes a conscious effort to provide your body with meals that support your desired level of fertility.

9. Be Adaptable and Flexible: Recognise that life is dynamic and that sustainable meal planning requires flexibility. Accept the ups and

downs of everyday life and give yourself permission to make changes while adhering to your fertility-related objectives. This advice ensures that meal planning stays a source of sustenance rather than worry by encouraging a pleasant and flexible attitude.

10. Seek Professional Advice: Take into Account Speaking with a dietitian or other medical specialist with expertise in infertility. Their knowledge can offer individualised recommendations for diet regimens that maximise your reproductive health, taking into account your particular requirements and objectives. This trick personalises your experience and makes your diet more focused on fertility work harder.

Allow these suggestions to assist you in crafting a gastronomic symphony that vibrates with harmony that enhances fertility as you immerse yourself in the art of meal preparation. Every meal turns into a planned action to boost ovulation, fuel your body, and embrace the

delicious convergence of fertility and flavour.
Welcome to a journey where meal preparation
transforms into a treasured custom, combining
aspiration and nutrition into each and every dish.

Breakfast Recipes

- **Nutrient-packed Smoothie Bowls**

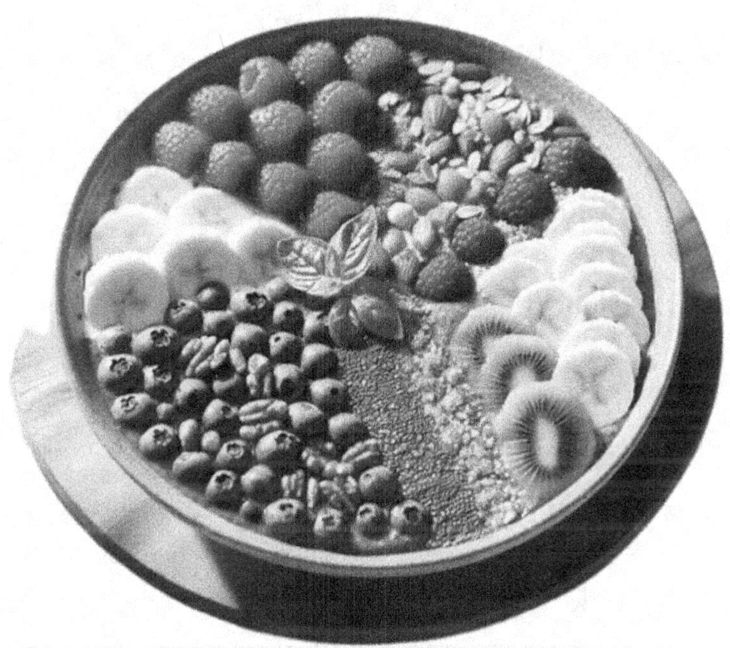

Ingredients:

- One cup of mixed berries, including raspberries, blueberries, and strawberries
- 1 frozen ripe banana
- half a cup of Greek yoghurt

- 1/4 cup almond milk, or your favourite kind of milk
- One spoonful of chia seeds
- One tablespoon of maple syrup or honey (optional; adds sweetness)
- Pumpkin seeds, granola, shredded coconut, and sliced kiwi are the toppings.

Preparation:

1. Blend together the frozen banana, Greek yoghurt, chia seeds, almond milk, mixed berries, and honey or maple syrup (if desired) in a blender.
2. The ingredients should be blended until a creamy, smooth consistency is reached. To make sure all of the ingredients are thoroughly combined, you might need to pause and scrape down the sides of the blender.
3. After blending, transfer the smoothie contents into a bowl.

Assembling the Bowl:

1. Place some sliced kiwis on top of the smoothie base to add more vitamins and a cool taste.
2. Scatter a substantial quantity of granola onto the bowl of smoothie. This gives it a nice crunch and an additional serving of fibre.
3. For a hint of natural sweetness and a tropical touch, add shredded coconut.
4. Add some extra nutrients and a source of healthy fats by finishing with a sprinkle of pumpkin seeds.

Nutritional Information(Approximate):

- 350 kcal of calories
- 15g of protein
- 60g of carbohydrates
- 12g of dietary fibre
- 30g of sugars
- 8g of fat
- Two grammes of saturated fat
- 250 mg of calcium

- Iron: 3 milligrammes

Servings: There is one serving per recipe. Adapt the amounts to your own tastes or the number of guests you're feeding.

Additional Tips:

1. Try varying the berry combinations to achieve a unique flavour profile.
2. Adjust the toppings to suit your tastes and what's in season.
3. For a dairy-free option, use unsweetened almond milk or other plant-based milk substitutes.
4. If you're trying to increase your protein consumption, feel free to add a scoop of protein powder to your smoothie bowl to increase its protein content.

Savour this nutrient-dense smoothie bowl as a tasty and stimulating way to start the day. It gives your body a variety of vital nutrients that support your overall health and fertility objectives.

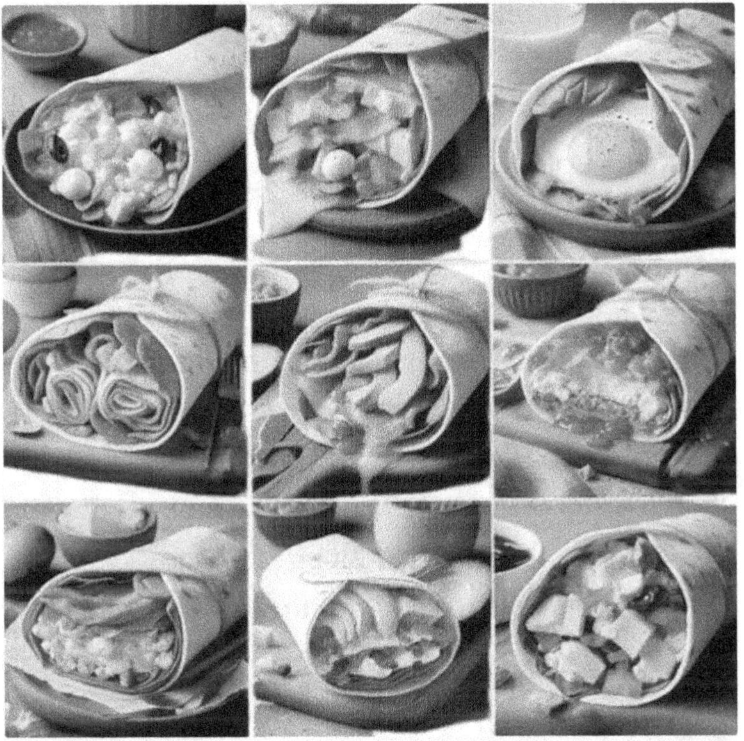

Ingredients:

1. Two large tortillas, either spinach or wholegrain
2. four big, beaten eggs
3. One cup of young spinach leaves

4. One medium-sized tomato, chopped; half an avocado, sliced; 1/4 cup of crumbled feta cheese
5. One tablespoon of olive oil
6. To taste, add salt and pepper.
7. Not required: For more flavour, use salsa or hot sauce.

Preparation:

1. To prepare the eggs, beat them in a bowl and season with pepper and salt.
2. In a skillet over medium heat, warm the olive oil.
3. Scramble the beaten eggs in the skillet until they are cooked to your desired consistency.

Put the Wraps Together:

1. To make the tortillas malleable, warm them for approximately 15 seconds in a dry skillet or microwave.

2. Spoon evenly between the two tortillas the
    scrambled eggs.

Incorporate New Ingredients:

1. Arrange a couple of baby spinach leaves,
    diced tomatoes, avocado slices, and
    crumbled feta cheese on top of each wrap.
2. Not required: Add Heat: Spoon salsa or
    drizzle with hot sauce over the filling for
    those who like a little kick of heat.

Put in a wrap and serve:

1. Each tortilla should be folded in half, then
    tightly rolled to create a wrap.
2. If necessary, fasten with a toothpick.
3. To make handling the wraps easier, cut
    them in half diagonally.

Estimated nutritional information:

- 400 kcal of calories
- 20g of protein

- 30g of carbohydrates
- 8g of dietary fibre
- 3g of sugars
- 25g of fat
- 7g of Saturated Fat
- 370 mg of cholesterol

Servings: Two energised breakfast wraps are produced from this recipe. Adapt the amounts to the number of servings required.

Additional Tips:

1. Try whole-grain or other types of wraps for more variation.
2. Tailor fillings to individual tastes; consider using sautéed mushrooms, bell peppers, or a sprinkling of your preferred herbs.
3. Prepare a large quantity of wraps and keep them chilled for an easy to grab-and-go breakfast.
4. These vivid veggie wraps are a tasty and healthy way to start the day, with a good

mix of healthy fats, protein, and colourful vegetables. The blend of tastes and textures in every mouthful guarantees a filling and healthy breakfast that supports your general health and provides you with energy for the entire morning.

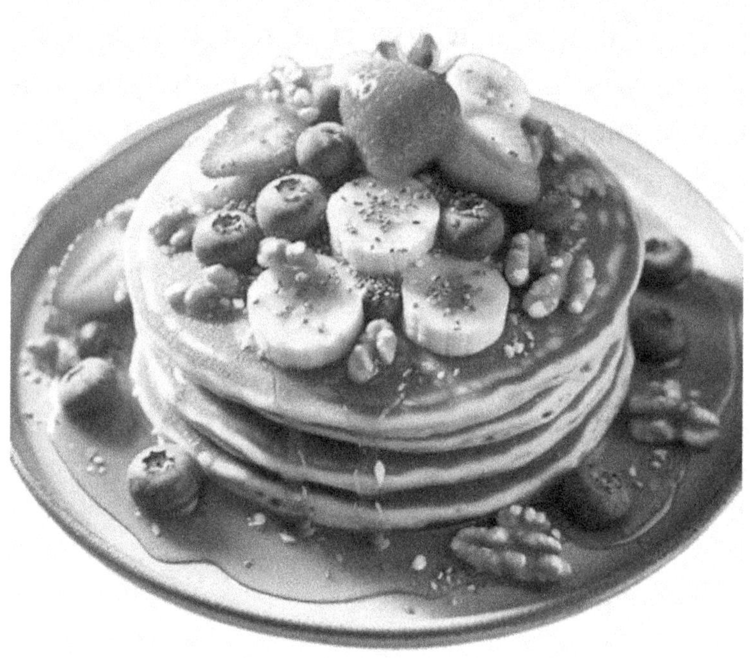

Ingredients:

- 1 cup oats (quick or rolled)
- 1 ripe banana
- 2 large eggs
- 1/2 cup Greek yogurt
- 1 teaspoon baking powder

- 1/2 teaspoon vanilla extract
- Pinch of salt
- Optional: 1-2 tablespoons honey or maple syrup for sweetness
- Cooking spray or a small amount of butter for the griddle

Preparation:

Blend the Batter:

1. In a blender or food processor, combine oats, banana, eggs, Greek yogurt, baking powder, vanilla extract, and a pinch of salt.
2. Blend until you achieve a smooth batter consistency. If the batter is too thick, you can add a splash of milk to reach the desired consistency.

Preheat the Griddle or Pan:

1. Heat a griddle or non-stick skillet over medium heat.
2. Lightly coat the surface with cooking spray or a small amount of butter.

Cook the Pancakes:

1. Pour 1/4 cup portions of batter onto the griddle, spacing them to allow for spreading.
2. Cook until bubbles form on the surface of the pancakes and the edges begin to set

Flip and Cook:

1. Gently flip the pancakes and cook the other side until golden brown and cooked through.

Serve Warm:

1. Remove the pancakes from the griddle and stack them on a plate.
2. Optional: Drizzle with honey or maple syrup for sweetness.

Nutritional Information (Approximate):

- Calories: 350 kcal
- Protein: 20g
- Carbohydrates: 45g

- Dietary Fiber: 5g
- Sugars: 10g
- Fat: 10g
- Saturated Fat: 3g
- Cholesterol: 190mg

Servings:

This recipe makes approximately 8 protein-rich pancakes. Adjust quantities based on your serving preferences.

Additional Tips:

1. Experiment with adding a scoop of your favorite protein powder to boost the protein content.
2. Top your pancakes with fresh berries, sliced bananas, or a dollop of Greek yogurt for added flavor and nutrition.
3. Consider making a larger batch and freezing extra pancakes for a quick and convenient breakfast option.

Lunch Ideas

- **Quinoa Salad with Fertility Boosting Veggies**

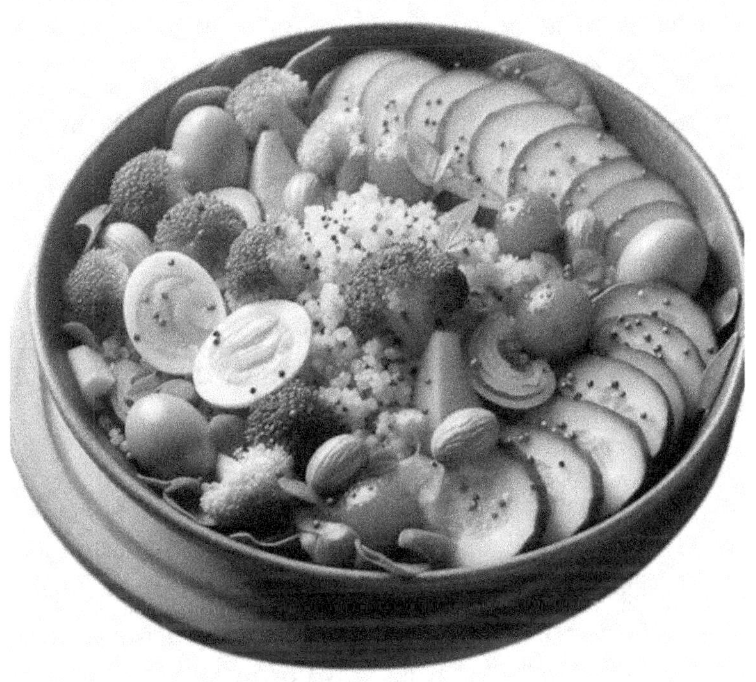

Ingredients:

- 1 cup quinoa, rinsed and cooked according to package instructions
- 2 cups mixed greens (spinach, kale, arugula)
- 1 cup cherry tomatoes, halved
- 1 cucumber, diced

- 1 bell pepper (any color), chopped
- 1/2 red onion, finely sliced
- 1/2 cup feta cheese, crumbled
- 1/4 cup Kalamata olives, pitted and sliced
- 1/4 cup extra-virgin olive oil
- 2 tablespoons balsamic vinegar
- 1 teaspoon Dijon mustard
- Salt and pepper to taste
- Optional: Grilled chicken or chickpeas for added protein

Preparation:

1. Rinse quinoa under cold water, then cook it according to package instructions. Allow it to cool completely.
2. In a small bowl, whisk together olive oil, balsamic vinegar, Dijon mustard, salt, and pepper. Set aside.
3. In a large salad bowl, combine the cooked quinoa, mixed greens, cherry tomatoes, cucumber, bell pepper, red onion, feta cheese, and Kalamata olives.
4. Toss the salad gently to distribute the ingredients evenly.

5. Drizzle the prepared dressing over the salad and toss again to coat the ingredients with the flavorful dressing.
6. **Optional Protein Boost:**
7. If desired, add grilled chicken slices or chickpeas to make the salad a more substantial and protein-rich meal.
8. Plate the quinoa salad, ensuring each serving has a colorful and nutritious mix of fertility-boosting veggies.
9. Garnish with additional feta cheese or olives if desired.

Nutritional Information (Approximate):

- Calories: 400 kcal
- Protein: 12g
- Carbohydrates: 45g
- Dietary Fiber: 8g
- Sugars: 5g
- Fat: 20g
- Saturated Fat: 5g
- Cholesterol: 15mg

Servings:

This recipe yields approximately 4 servings. Adjust quantities based on your serving preferences or add more protein for a heartier meal.

Additional Tips:

1. Experiment with different veggies based on seasonal availability.
2. Make the salad ahead of time and refrigerate, allowing flavors to meld for an even tastier experience.
3. Customize the dressing by adding herbs like fresh basil or oregano for an extra burst of flavor.

- **Grilled Chicken and Avacado Wrap**

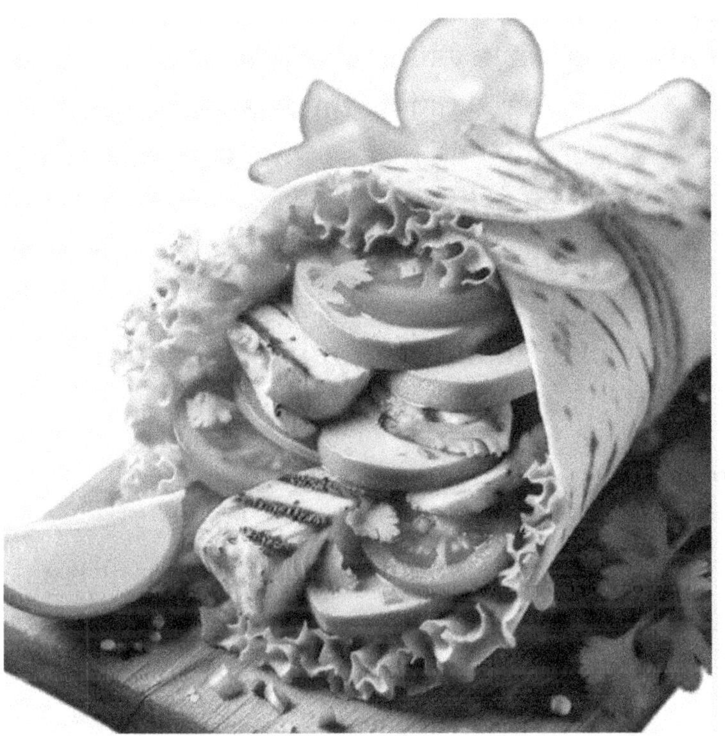

Ingredients:

- 2 boneless, skinless chicken breasts
- 1 tablespoon olive oil
- 1 teaspoon cumin
- 1 teaspoon paprika
- Salt and pepper to taste

- 4 whole-grain or spinach tortillas
- 1 ripe avocado, sliced
- 1 cup cherry tomatoes, halved
- 1/2 cup red onion, thinly sliced
- 1 cup mixed greens (arugula, spinach, or your choice)
- 1/4 cup Greek yogurt or your favorite dressing
- Optional: Squeeze of lime for added freshness

Preparation:

1. In a bowl, mix olive oil, cumin, paprika, salt, and pepper.
2. Coat the chicken breasts with the spice mixture.
3. Grill the chicken on medium-high heat until fully cooked, approximately 6-8 minutes per side. Allow it to rest before slicing.
4. Warm the tortillas on a dry skillet or microwave for about 15 seconds to make them pliable.

5. Lay out each tortilla and place sliced grilled chicken down the center.
6. Top the chicken with avocado slices, cherry tomatoes, red onion, and mixed greens.
7. Spoon Greek yogurt or your preferred dressing over the ingredients. A squeeze of lime adds a zesty kick.
8. Fold in the sides of each tortilla and roll it up tightly to form a wrap.
9. Slice the wraps in half diagonally for easy serving.

Nutritional Information (Approximate):

- Calories: 400 kcal
- Protein: 30g
- Carbohydrates: 30g
- Dietary Fiber: 8g
- Sugars: 4g
- Fat: 18g
- Saturated Fat: 3g
- Cholesterol: 70mg

Servings:

This recipe makes approximately 4 grilled chicken and avocado wraps. Adjust quantities based on your serving preferences.

Additional Tips:

1. Marinate the chicken in the spice mixture for extra flavor; let it sit in the refrigerator for at least 30 minutes before grilling.
2. Customize the veggies based on personal preferences—try adding bell peppers, cucumbers, or shredded carrots.
3. For a spicy kick, add a dash of hot sauce or sprinkle chili flakes over the grilled chicken before wrapping.

- **Lentil Soup for Balanced Nutrition**

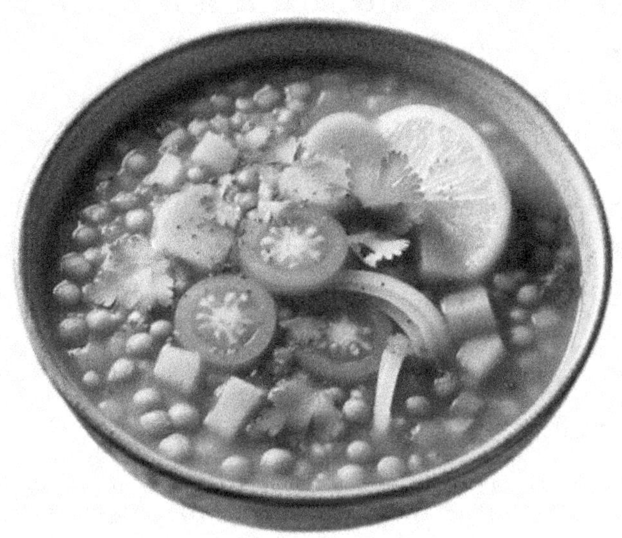

Ingredients:

- 1 cup dried green or brown lentils, rinsed
- 1 large onion, finely chopped
- 2 carrots, diced
- 2 celery stalks, diced
- 3 cloves garlic, minced

- 1 can (14 oz) diced tomatoes, undrained
- 6 cups vegetable or chicken broth
- 1 teaspoon ground cumin
- 1 teaspoon ground coriander
- 1/2 teaspoon smoked paprika
- 1 bay leaf
- Salt and pepper to taste
- 2 cups fresh spinach, chopped
- Juice of one lemon
- Olive oil for drizzling (optional)
- Fresh parsley for garnish (optional)

Preparation:

1. In a large pot, heat olive oil over medium heat.Add chopped onion, carrots, and celery.
2. Sauté until the vegetables are softened.
3. Stir in minced garlic, cumin, coriander, smoked paprika, salt, and pepper.
4. Add rinsed lentils to the pot and coat them with the aromatic vegetables and spices.
5. Pour in diced tomatoes (with their juice) and vegetable or chicken broth.
6. Add a bay leaf for extra flavor.

7. Bring the soup to a boil, then reduce heat and let it simmer until lentils are tender, usually 20-25 minutes.
8. Stir in fresh chopped spinach and let it wilt into the soup.
9. Squeeze in the juice of one lemon for brightness and a touch of acidity.
10. Taste and adjust the seasoning with additional salt and pepper if needed.
11. Discard the bay leaf before serving.
12. Drizzle olive oil over each serving for richness.
13. Garnish with fresh parsley for a burst of freshness.

Nutritional Information (Approximate):

- Calories: 250 kcal
- Protein: 15g
- Carbohydrates: 40g
- Dietary Fiber: 15g
- Sugars: 6g
- Fat: 3g
- Saturated Fat: 0.5g
- Cholesterol: 0mg

Servings:

This recipe makes approximately 6 servings. Adjust quantities based on your preferences or store leftovers for later consumption.

Additional Tips:

1. Experiment with different lentil varieties for varied textures and flavors.
2. Consider adding a pinch of red pepper flakes for a hint of heat.

Serve the lentil soup with a side of whole-grain bread for a complete and satisfying meal.

Dinner Delights

- **Salmon with Roasted Sweet Potatoes**

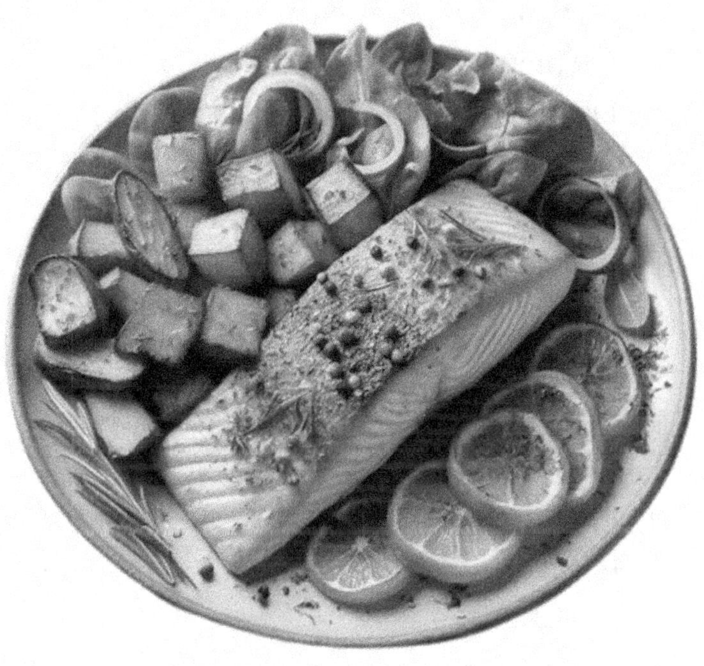

Ingredients:

- 4 salmon fillets
- 4 medium-sized sweet potatoes, peeled and diced

- 2 tablespoons olive oil
- 1 teaspoon garlic powder
- 1 teaspoon smoked paprika
- 1 teaspoon dried thyme
- Salt and pepper to taste
- 1 lemon, sliced
- Fresh parsley for garnish (optional)

Preparation:

1. Preheat the oven to 400°F (200°C).
2. Place salmon fillets on a lined baking sheet.
3. Drizzle with olive oil and season with garlic powder, smoked paprika, dried thyme, salt, and pepper.
4. Place lemon slices on top of the salmon fillets.
5. Toss diced sweet potatoes with olive oil, salt, and pepper.
6. Spread them in a single layer on a separate baking sheet.
7. Roast both the salmon and sweet potatoes in the preheated oven.

8. Bake the sweet potatoes for about 25-30 minutes or until tender and slightly caramelized.
9. Bake the salmon for approximately 15-20 minutes or until it flakes easily with a fork.
10. Arrange roasted sweet potatoes on plates.
11. Top with a salmon fillet and garnish with fresh parsley if desired.

Nutritional Information (Approximate):

- Calories: 400 kcal
- Protein: 30g
- Carbohydrates: 30g
- Dietary Fiber: 5g
- Sugars: 6g
- Fat: 20g
- Saturated Fat: 3g
- Cholesterol: 80mg

Servings:

This recipe makes approximately 4 servings.
Adjust quantities based on your preferences or
the number of diners.

Additional Tips:

1. For added flavor, consider marinating the
   salmon in a mix of lemon juice, olive oil,
   and herbs before baking.
2. Customize the sweet potatoes with your
   preferred spices or add a touch of
   cinnamon for sweetness.
3. Serve with a side of steamed vegetables or
   a green salad for a well-rounded dinner.

- **Vegetarian Stir-Fry with Tofu**

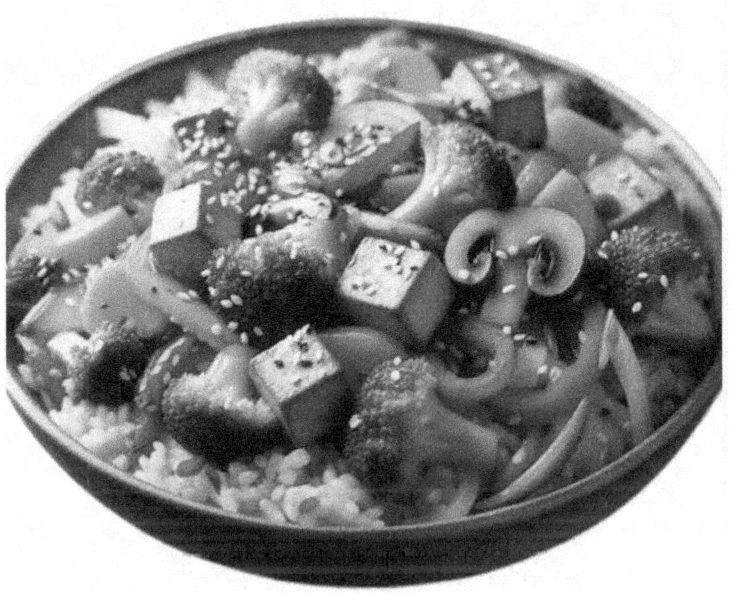

Ingredients:

- 1 block (14 oz) extra-firm tofu, pressed
  and cubed
- 3 tablespoons soy sauce (low-sodium)
- 2 tablespoons sesame oil
- 1 tablespoon rice vinegar
- 1 tablespoon maple syrup or agave nectar
- 1 tablespoon cornstarch

- 2 tablespoons vegetable oil
- 1 tablespoon ginger, minced
- 3 cloves garlic, minced
- 1 bell pepper, thinly sliced
- 1 carrot, julienned
- 1 cup broccoli florets
- 1 cup snap peas, trimmed
- 1 cup sliced mushrooms
- 4 green onions, sliced
- Sesame seeds for garnish
- Cooked brown rice or quinoa for serving

Preparation:

1. Press the tofu to remove excess water, then cut it into bite-sized cubes.
2. In a bowl, whisk together soy sauce, sesame oil, rice vinegar, maple syrup (or agave nectar), and cornstarch to create the marinade.
3. Add tofu cubes to the marinade, ensuring they are well-coated. Allow it to marinate for at least 15-20 minutes.
4. Heat vegetable oil in a wok or large skillet over medium-high heat.

5. Add marinated tofu cubes and cook until they are golden brown and crispy. Remove from the pan and set aside.
6. In the same pan, add a bit more oil if needed.
7. Sauté ginger and garlic until fragrant.
8. Add bell pepper, carrot, broccoli, snap peas, and mushrooms. Stir-fry until the vegetables are crisp-tender.
9. Return the cooked tofu to the pan, combining it with the sautéed vegetables.
10. Stir in sliced green onions.
11. Garnish with sesame seeds.
12. Serve the vegetarian stir-fry over cooked brown rice or quinoa.

Nutritional Information (Approximate):

- Calories: 350 kcal
- Protein: 20g
- Carbohydrates: 30g
- Dietary Fiber: 6g
- Sugars: 8g
- Fat: 18g
- Saturated Fat: 2g

- Cholesterol: 0mg

Servings:

This recipe makes approximately 4 servings. Adjust quantities based on your preferences or the number of diners.

Additional Tips:

1. Add a kick of heat with red pepper flakes or sriracha sauce.
2. Experiment with different vegetables based on your preferences or what's in season.
3. For extra crunch, sprinkle chopped peanuts or cashews over the stir-fry before serving.

- **Whole Grain Pasta Primavera**

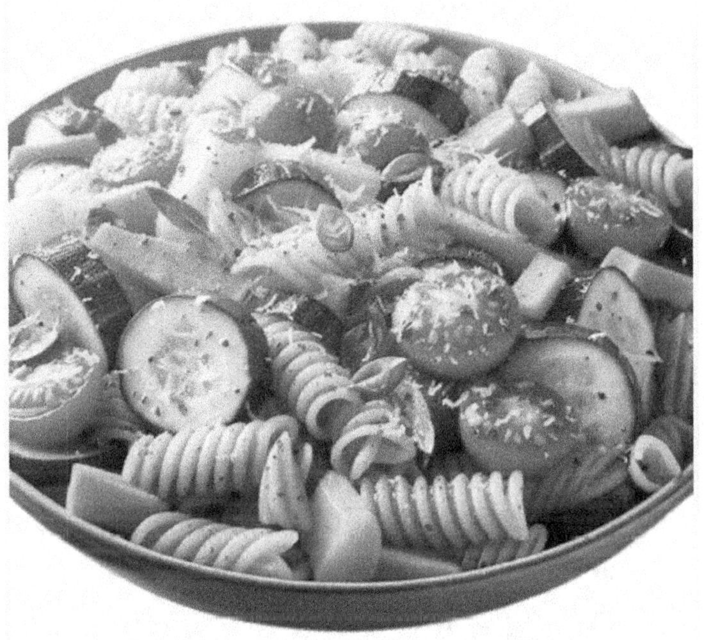

Ingredients:

- 8 oz whole grain pasta (spaghetti or your choice)
- 2 tablespoons olive oil
- 3 cloves garlic, minced
- 1 onion, thinly sliced
- 1 bell pepper, julienned

- 1 zucchini, sliced
- 1 yellow squash, sliced
- 1 cup cherry tomatoes, halved
- 1 cup broccoli florets
- 1 cup baby spinach leaves
- 1/2 cup grated Parmesan cheese
- 1/4 cup fresh basil, chopped
- Salt and pepper to taste
- Red pepper flakes for optional heat

Preparation:

- Boil the whole grain pasta according to package instructions until al dente. Drain and set aside.
- In a large skillet, heat olive oil over medium heat.
- Sauté minced garlic until fragrant, then add sliced onions. Cook until onions are translucent.
- Add bell pepper, zucchini, yellow squash, cherry tomatoes, and broccoli to the skillet.
- Sauté until the vegetables are crisp-tender, maintaining their vibrant colors.

- Add the cooked whole grain pasta to the skillet, tossing it with the sautéed vegetables.
- Stir in baby spinach, allowing it to wilt.
- Sprinkle grated Parmesan cheese over the pasta and vegetables.
- Season with salt and pepper to taste. Add red pepper flakes if you desire a bit of heat.
- Garnish the Pasta Primavera with fresh chopped basil.
- Serve warm, with additional Parmesan cheese on the side if desired.

Nutritional Information (Approximate):

- Calories: 400 kcal
- Protein: 15g
- Carbohydrates: 60g
- Dietary Fiber: 10g
- Sugars: 6g
- Fat: 12g
- Saturated Fat: 3g
- Cholesterol: 10mg

Servings:

This recipe makes approximately 4 servings. Adjust quantities based on your preferences or the number of diners.

Additional Tips:

1. Experiment with different whole grain pasta varieties like whole wheat or quinoa pasta.
2. Customize the vegetables based on seasonal availability or personal preferences.
3. Drizzle extra olive oil or a squeeze of lemon juice over the pasta before serving for added flavor.

Snacks

- **Fertility-Boosting Trail Mix**

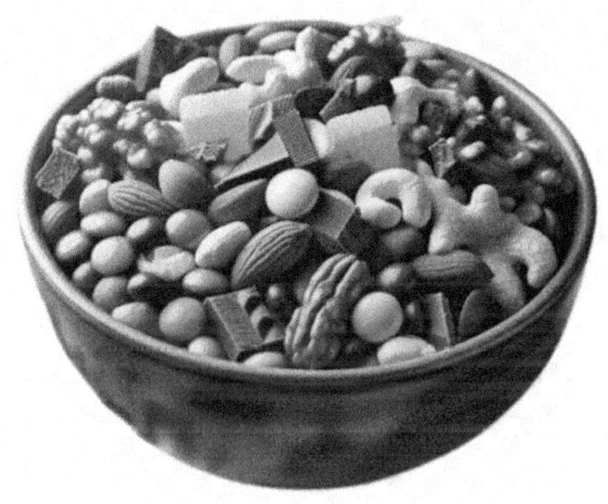

Ingredients:

- 1 cup raw almonds

- 1 cup walnuts
- 1/2 cup pumpkin seeds
- 1/2 cup dried goji berries
- 1/2 cup dried apricots, chopped
- 1/2 cup dark chocolate chips (at least 70% cocoa)
- 1/2 teaspoon cinnamon
- Pinch of sea salt

Preparation:

1. In a dry skillet, lightly toast almonds, walnuts, and pumpkin seeds over medium heat. Stir occasionally to prevent burning. Once fragrant, remove from heat and let them cool.
2. In a large bowl, combine the toasted nuts and seeds with dried goji berries, chopped dried apricots, and dark chocolate chips.
3. Sprinkle cinnamon over the mixture for a warm and aromatic touch.
4. Add a pinch of sea salt to enhance the flavors.
5. Gently toss all the ingredients together until they are evenly distributed.

6. Transfer the fertility-boosting trail mix to an airtight container for storage.

Nutritional Information (Approximate):

- Calories: 200 kcal (per 1/4 cup serving)
- Protein: 5g
- Carbohydrates: 15g
- Dietary Fiber: 3g
- Sugars: 7g
- Fat: 15g
- Saturated Fat: 3g

Servings:

This recipe makes approximately 4 cups of trail mix. Adjust quantities based on your preferences.

Additional Tips:

1. Customize the trail mix by adding other fertility-friendly ingredients such as chia seeds or dried cherries.
2. Portion the trail mix into small snack bags for convenient and controlled servings.

3. Enjoy this fertility-boosting trail mix as a snack between meals or a quick energy boost during the day.

- **Greek Yogurt Parfait**

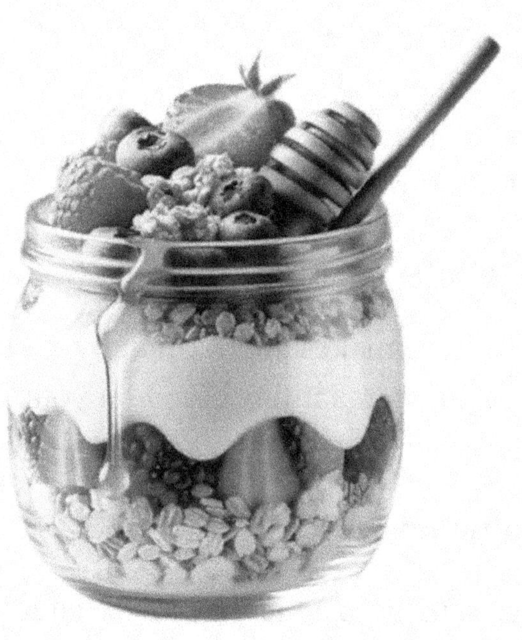

Ingredients:

- 1 cup Greek yogurt (unsweetened)
- 1/2 cup granola (choose a low-sugar or homemade option)
- 1/2 cup mixed berries (strawberries, blueberries, raspberries)
- 1 tablespoon honey or maple syrup (optional, for sweetness)
- 1 tablespoon chia seeds
- 1/4 cup sliced almonds
- Fresh mint leaves for garnish (optional)

Preparation:

1. In a glass or bowl, start with a layer of Greek yogurt as the base.
2. Sprinkle a layer of granola over the Greek yogurt. This provides a satisfying crunch and additional fiber.
3. Add a generous layer of mixed berries, distributing them evenly for a burst of natural sweetness and antioxidants.
4. If you prefer extra sweetness, drizzle honey or maple syrup over the berries.

5. Sprinkle chia seeds and sliced almonds over the parfait, adding a boost of omega-3 fatty acids and crunch.
6. Repeat the layering process until you reach the top of the glass or bowl.
7. Optionally, garnish the top with fresh mint leaves for a refreshing touch.

Nutritional Information (Approximate):

- Calories: 350 kcal
- Protein: 20g
- Carbohydrates: 40g
- Dietary Fiber: 8g
- Sugars: 15g
- Fat: 15g
- Saturated Fat: 3g

Servings:

This recipe makes one Greek Yogurt Parfait. Adjust quantities based on your preferences.

Additional Tips:

1. Experiment with different fruits and nuts
   based on your taste preferences or
   seasonal availability.
2. Consider using flavored Greek yogurt for
   added variety.
3. Prepare the parfait ahead of time, keeping
   it refrigerated until you're ready to enjoy.

- **Homemade Energy Bars**

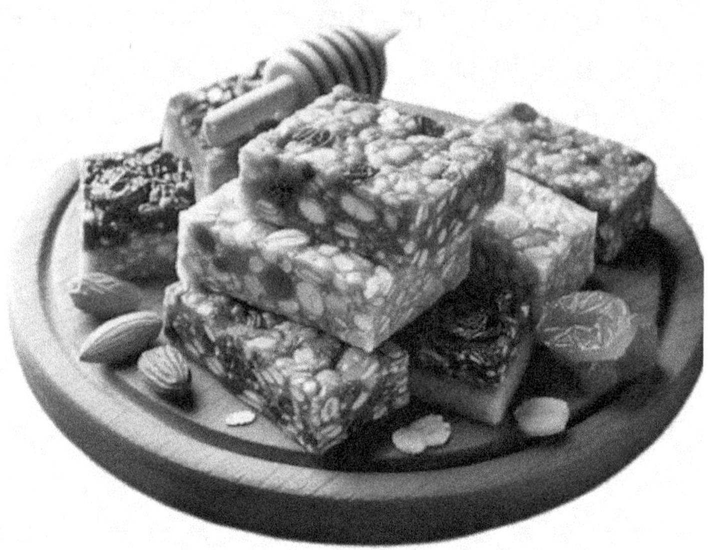

Ingredients:

- 1 cup rolled oats
- 1/2 cup almonds, chopped
- 1/4 cup walnuts, chopped
- 1/4 cup chia seeds

- 1/2 cup dried fruits (apricots, dates, raisins), chopped
- 1/4 cup almond butter
- 1/4 cup honey or maple syrup
- 1 teaspoon vanilla extract
- 1/2 teaspoon cinnamon
- Pinch of salt

Preparation:

1. In a large bowl, combine rolled oats, chopped almonds, walnuts, chia seeds, and dried fruits.
2. In a small saucepan over low heat, warm the almond butter and honey (or maple syrup) until they are easily mixable. Stir frequently.
3. Pour the warmed almond butter and honey (or maple syrup) mixture over the dry ingredients.
4. Add vanilla extract, cinnamon, and a pinch of salt.
5. Mix well until all ingredients are thoroughly combined.

6. Line a square or rectangular pan with
   parchment paper.
7. Transfer the mixture into the pan and
   press it down firmly to create an even
   layer.
8. Place the pan in the refrigerator for at least
   2 hours, allowing the mixture to set.
9. Once the mixture has hardened, remove it
   from the refrigerator.
10. Use a sharp knife to cut it into individual
    energy bars.
11. Store the homemade energy bars in an
    airtight container in the refrigerator for
    freshness.

Nutritional Information (Approximate):

- Calories: 200 kcal (per bar)
- Protein: 5g
- Carbohydrates: 20g
- Dietary Fiber: 4g
- Sugars: 10g
- Fat: 12g
- Saturated Fat: 1g

Servings:

This recipe makes approximately 8-10 homemade energy bars. Adjust quantities based on your preferences.

Additional Tips:

1. Customize the recipe by adding your favorite nuts, seeds, or dried fruits.
2. Experiment with different nut butters for varied flavors.
3. Wrap individual bars in parchment paper for a convenient grab-and-go snack.

Desserts with a Purpose

- **Berry Bliss Smoothie Pops**

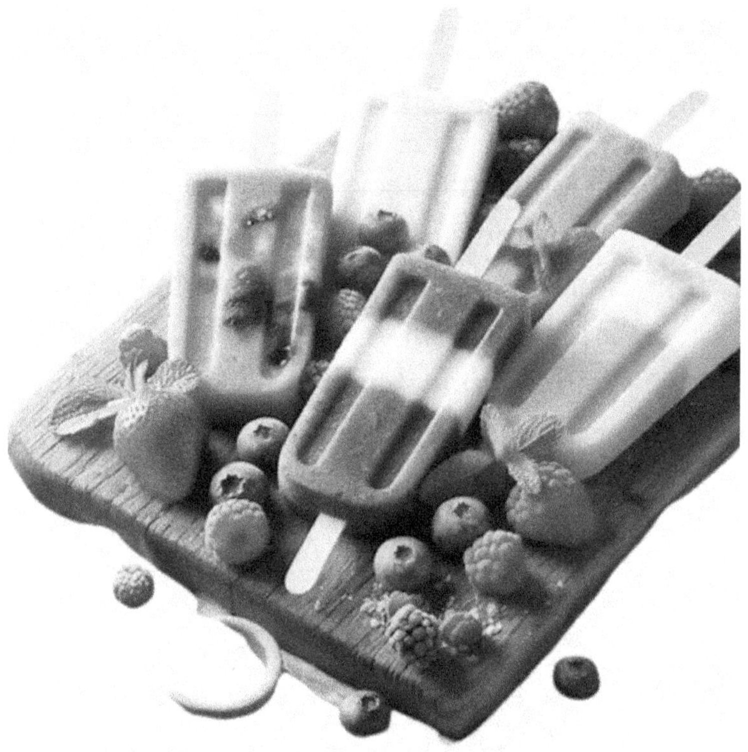

Ingredients:

- 1 cup mixed berries (strawberries, blueberries, raspberries)

- 1 banana, peeled
- 1 cup Greek yogurt (unsweetened)
- 2 tablespoons honey or maple syrup
- 1/2 teaspoon vanilla extract
- 1/4 cup chia seeds
- 1/2 cup granola (optional, for added crunch)

Preparation:

1. In a blender, combine mixed berries, peeled banana, Greek yogurt, honey (or maple syrup), and vanilla extract.
2. Blend until you achieve a smooth and creamy consistency.
3. Stir in chia seeds into the smoothie mixture, ensuring they are evenly distributed. Chia seeds will add texture and boost the nutritional content.
4. Pour the berry and chia seed mixture into popsicle molds, leaving a little space at the top for expansion.
5. If using, sprinkle granola into each mold for added crunch.

6. Place popsicle sticks into each mold, ensuring they are centered.
7. Place the popsicle molds in the freezer and let them freeze for at least 4-6 hours or until solid.
8. Once the popsicles are completely frozen, run the molds under warm water for a few seconds to loosen the popsicles.
9. Gently remove the popsicles from the molds and serve.

Nutritional Information (Approximate):

- Calories: 120 kcal (per popsicle)
- Protein: 4g
- Carbohydrates: 20g
- Dietary Fiber: 5g
- Sugars: 10g
- Fat: 3g
- Saturated Fat: 1g

Servings:

This recipe makes approximately 6 Berry Bliss Smoothie Pops. Adjust quantities based on your preferences.

Additional Tips:

1. Experiment with different berry combinations or add a handful of spinach for added nutrients.
2. Customize sweetness by adjusting the amount of honey or maple syrup.
3. Before serving, roll the popsicles in shredded coconut for a delightful touch.

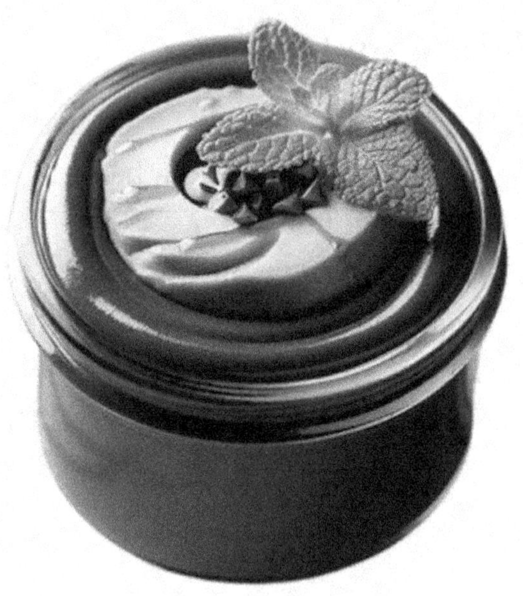

Ingredients:

- 2 ripe avocados, peeled and pitted
- 1/2 cup dark chocolate chips (at least 70% cocoa)
- 1/4 cup unsweetened cocoa powder

- 1/4 cup maple syrup or honey
- 1 teaspoon vanilla extract
- Pinch of salt
- Fresh berries for garnish (optional)
- Whipped coconut cream for topping (optional)

Preparation:

1. In a heatproof bowl, melt dark chocolate chips using a double boiler or microwave in short intervals, stirring until smooth.
2. In a blender or food processor, combine ripe avocados, melted dark chocolate, unsweetened cocoa powder, maple syrup (or honey), vanilla extract, and a pinch of salt.
3. Blend until you achieve a creamy and velvety mousse consistency.
4. Transfer the chocolate avocado mousse into individual serving glasses or bowls.
5. Chill in the refrigerator for at least 1-2 hours to allow the mousse to set.

6. Before serving, garnish with fresh berries
   and a dollop of whipped coconut cream if
   desired.

Nutritional Information (Approximate):

- Calories: 200 kcal (per serving)
- Protein: 3g
- Carbohydrates: 20g
- Dietary Fiber: 8g
- Sugars: 10g
- Fat: 15g
- Saturated Fat: 5g

Servings:

This recipe makes approximately 4 servings of
Dark Chocolate Avocado Mousse. Adjust
quantities based on your preferences.

Additional Tips:

1. Experiment with flavored dark chocolate
   or add a hint of espresso for an extra depth
   of flavor.

2. Adjust sweetness by adding more or less maple syrup/honey according to taste.
3. Serve the mousse with a sprinkle of chopped nuts for added crunch.

- **Fruit Salad with Mint**

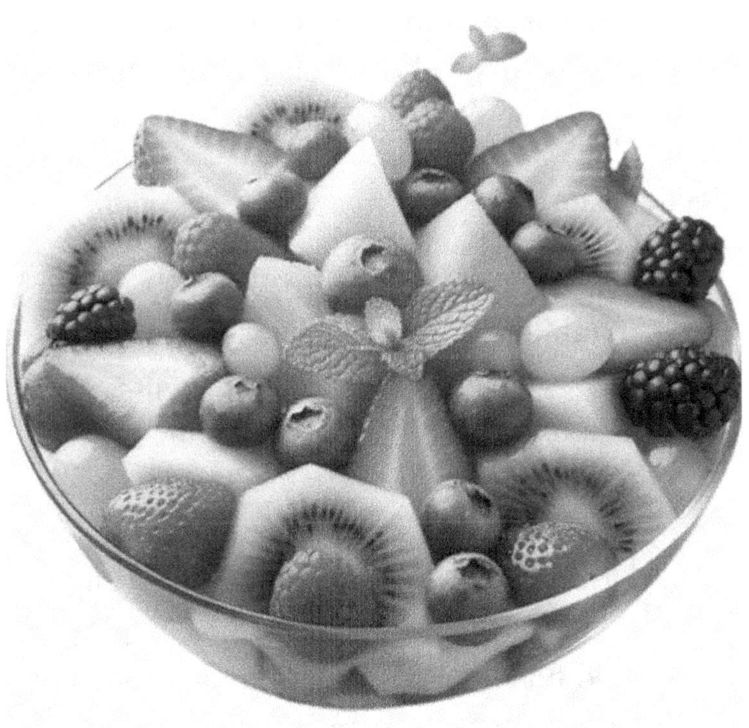

Ingredients:

- 2 cups fresh strawberries, hulled and halved
- 1 cup fresh blueberries
- 1 cup fresh pineapple, diced
- 1 cup green grapes, halved
- 1 mango, peeled, pitted, and diced
- 1 tablespoon fresh lime juice
- 2 tablespoons honey or maple syrup
- Fresh mint leaves for garnish

Preparation:

1. Wash and prepare all the fruits as directed – hull and halve strawberries, dice pineapple and mango, halve grapes.
2. In a large mixing bowl, combine the prepared strawberries, blueberries, pineapple, grapes, and mango.
3. Drizzle fresh lime juice over the fruit salad to enhance flavors.
4. Add honey or maple syrup for a touch of sweetness. Adjust according to taste.

5. Gently toss the fruit salad to ensure the fruits are evenly coated with lime juice and sweetener.
6. For optimal freshness, refrigerate the fruit salad for at least 30 minutes before serving.
7. Just before serving, sprinkle fresh mint leaves over the fruit salad for a burst of aromatic freshness.

Nutritional Information (Approximate):

- Calories: 150 kcal (per serving)
- Protein: 2g
- Carbohydrates: 38g
- Dietary Fiber: 5g
- Sugars: 30g
- Fat: 1g
- Saturated Fat: 0g

Servings:

This recipe makes approximately 4 servings of Fruit Salad with Mint. Adjust quantities based on your preferences.

Additional Tips:

1. Add a splash of orange juice for an extra citrusy flavor.
2. Experiment with different seasonal fruits for variety.
3. Serve the fruit salad in individual bowls or as a refreshing side dish for brunch or dessert.

Lifestyle Tips for Fertility

Keep Your Diet Balanced:
Eat a diet full of fruits, vegetables, whole grains, lean meats, and healthy fats. Sufficient food intake promotes both general health and fertility.

Remain Hydrated:
To stay hydrated, sip lots of water throughout the day. Drinking enough water is essential for good health in general, especially reproductive health.

Regular Exercise:
To maintain a healthy weight and encourage blood circulation, partake in regular physical activity. Try to get in at least 150 minutes a week of moderate-to-intense activity.

Handle stress by exercising:
Engaging in stress-relieving exercises like yoga, meditation, or deep breathing. Infertility can be adversely affected by prolonged stress, therefore learning how to relax is crucial.

Sufficient Sleep:
 Make sure you receive seven to nine hours of good sleep every night. Hormone balance and general reproductive health depend on sleep.

Moderate Alcohol and Caffeine Consumption: Restrict your intake of alcohol and caffeine. Moderate consumption of alcohol and caffeine is recommended as excessive consumption of these substances may impact fertility.

Give Up Smoking:
 It is strongly advised that smokers give up. There is evidence linking smoking to lower fertility in both men and women.

Keep Your Weight in Check:
 Aim for a healthy weight by eating a balanced diet and getting frequent exercise. Conditions involving underweight or overweight people might affect fertility.

Recognise Menstrual Cycle:

Become acquainted with your ovulation and menstrual cycles. This information can aid in maximising the time of conception.

Reduce Exposure to Hazardous Chemicals and Toxins in the Environment:
Reduce your exposure to hazardous chemicals and toxins in your surroundings, such as pollution, pesticides, and some cleaning supplies.

Take Prenatal Supplements Into Consideration:
If you're trying to get pregnant, you might want to think about taking prenatal vitamins that include folic acid and other vital nutrients.

Communication with Your Partner:
Continue to have frank and open discussions about your infertility journey with your partner. Offer emotional support to one another and, if necessary, seek professional assistance.

Frequent Check-ups: Arrange for routine medical examinations to treat any underlying health issues that may impact fertility.

Become Knowledgeable:
Continue to learn about reproductive health and fertility. Knowing the natural processes of your body might help you become more powerful during the conception process.

Seek Expert Advice:
 Speak with a fertility doctor if conception is taking longer than anticipated. Potential problems can be found and addressed early on.

These lifestyle suggestions can support a comprehensive approach to fertility, enhancing general health and raising the likelihood of a healthy conception journey.

Weekly Meal Plan

Week 1

Day 1: Balanced Start

Breakfast

- Nutrient-packed Smoothie Bowl with mixed berries, Greek yogurt, chia seeds, and a sprinkle of granola.

Lunch

- Quinoa Salad with Fertility-Boosting Veggies: Quinoa, cherry tomatoes, cucumbers, avocados, and a light lemon vinaigrette.

Dinner

- Grilled Salmon with Roasted Sweet Potatoes: A protein-rich dinner paired with sweet potatoes for complex carbs.

Day 2: Energizing Choices

Breakfast

- Energizing Breakfast Wraps: Whole-grain tortillas filled with scrambled eggs, spinach, and a touch of salsa.

Lunch

- Vegetarian Stir-Fry with Tofu: A colorful mix of tofu, broccoli, bell peppers, and snap peas stir-fried in a savory sauce.

Dinner

- Protein-rich Pancakes: Whole grain pancakes topped with Greek yogurt, fresh berries, and a drizzle of honey.

Day 3: Wholesome Indulgence

Breakfast

- Dark Chocolate Avocado Mousse: A decadent yet healthy breakfast option with avocados, dark chocolate, and a touch of sweetness.

Lunch

- Lentil Soup for Balanced Nutrition: A hearty and nutritious soup with green lentils, vegetables, and aromatic spices.

Dinner

- Whole Grain Pasta Primavera: A colorful pasta dish loaded with whole-grain goodness and a variety of fresh vegetables.

Day 4: Nourishing Options

Breakfast

- Greek Yogurt Parfait: Layers of Greek yogurt, granola, mixed berries, and a drizzle of honey.

Lunch

- Grilled Chicken and Avocado Wrap: A satisfying wrap with grilled chicken, avocado, lettuce, and a light dressing.

Dinner

- Salmon with Quinoa and Steamed Vegetables: A complete meal with omega-3-rich salmon, quinoa, and a medley of steamed veggies.

Day 5: Plant-Powered Delight

Breakfast

- Whole Grain Toast with Nut Butter and Sliced Banana: A quick and energizing breakfast option.

Lunch

- Quinoa and Black Bean Bowl: A plant-powered bowl with quinoa, black beans, corn, tomatoes, and a zesty lime dressing.

Dinner

- Lentil Stuffed Bell Peppers: Bell peppers filled with a mixture of lentils, vegetables, and herbs, baked to perfection.

Day 6: Fresh and Flavorful

Breakfast

- Fertility-Boosting Trail Mix: A handful of nuts, seeds, and dried fruits for a quick and nourishing morning snack.

Lunch

- Homemade Energy Bars: A wholesome blend of oats, nuts, dried fruits, and natural sweeteners.

Dinner

- Vegetable Stir-Fry with Brown Rice: A colorful stir-fry with an assortment of vegetables served over nutrient-rich brown rice.

Day 7: Sweet & Simple

Breakfast

- Overnight Oats with Almond Milk and Berries: Prepare the night before for a convenient and nutritious breakfast.

Lunch

- Spinach and Chickpea Salad: A refreshing salad with spinach, chickpeas, cherry tomatoes, and a lemony dressing.

Dinner

- Fruit Salad with Mint: A light and refreshing dessert-like dinner option with a variety of fresh fruits and a hint of mint.

Week 2

Day 8: Comforting Choices

Breakfast

- Greek Yogurt with Honey and Mixed Nuts: A simple yet satisfying combination for a nutritious start.

Lunch

- Quinoa and Vegetable Soup: A hearty
  soup with quinoa, a variety of vegetables,
  and flavorful broth.

Dinner

- Baked Cod with Lemon and Herbs: Light
  and flavorful baked cod paired with a side
  of steamed broccoli.

Day 9: Vibrant & Nutrient-Rich

Breakfast

- Berry Bliss Smoothie Pops: A fun and
  fruity way to kickstart the day with a
  homemade smoothie popsicle.

Lunch

- Mediterranean Chickpea Salad: A vibrant
  salad with chickpeas, cherry tomatoes,
  cucumbers, olives, and feta cheese.

Dinner

- Grilled Veggie and Hummus Wrap: A satisfying wrap filled with grilled vegetables and a generous spread of hummus.

Day 10: Sweet & Savory Combination

Breakfast

- Dark Chocolate Avocado Toast: Whole-grain toast topped with mashed avocado and a sprinkle of dark chocolate chips.

Lunch

- Quinoa and Roasted Vegetable Bowl: A nourishing bowl featuring quinoa, roasted vegetables, and a drizzle of balsamic glaze.

Dinner

- Chicken and Vegetable Skewers: Marinated and grilled chicken skewers with colorful bell peppers and onions.

Day 11: Nutrient-Packed Fusion

Breakfast

- Acai Bowl with Mixed Berries and Coconut Flakes: A refreshing and antioxidant-rich breakfast bowl.

Lunch

- Lentil and Sweet Potato Curry: A flavorful curry with lentils, sweet potatoes, and aromatic spices served over brown rice.

Dinner

- Shrimp and Avocado Salad: A light and protein-packed salad with shrimp, avocado, mixed greens, and a citrusy dressing.

Day 12: Satisfying & Wholesome

Breakfast

- Banana Nut Overnight Oats: Overnight oats with sliced bananas, chopped nuts, and a drizzle of maple syrup.

Lunch

- Spinach and Feta Stuffed Chicken Breast: Baked chicken breasts stuffed with a spinach and feta cheese filling.

Dinner

- Quinoa-Stuffed Bell Peppers: Bell peppers filled with a mixture of quinoa, black beans, corn, and spices.

Day 13: Balanced & Energizing

Breakfast

- Veggie Omelette with Whole Grain Toast: A nutrient-packed omelette filled with colorful vegetables.

Lunch

- Chickpea and Spinach Wrap: A satisfying wrap with chickpeas, spinach, tomatoes, and a light dressing.

Dinner

- Baked Turkey Meatballs with Zucchini Noodles: Lean turkey meatballs baked to perfection, served over zucchini noodles.

Day 14: Finishing Strong

Breakfast

- Mixed Berry and Spinach Smoothie: A refreshing smoothie with mixed berries, spinach, Greek yogurt, and a touch of honey.

Lunch

- Quinoa and Black Bean Stuffed Sweet Potatoes: Baked sweet potatoes filled with a hearty mixture of quinoa and black beans.

Dinner

- Grilled Vegetable and Quinoa Salad: A light and colorful salad featuring grilled vegetables, quinoa, and a lemon herb dressing.

Week 3

Day 15: Celebrating Variety

Breakfast

- Protein-Packed Breakfast Burrito: A satisfying burrito filled with scrambled eggs, black beans, avocado, and salsa.

Lunch

- Asian-Inspired Tofu and Vegetable Stir-Fry: Stir-fried tofu with a colorful mix of vegetables and a sesame-ginger sauce.

Dinner

- Baked Chicken with Quinoa and
  Asparagus: Tender baked chicken served
  with quinoa and roasted asparagus.

Day 16: Wholesome & Hearty

Breakfast

- Overnight Chia Seed Pudding: Chia seeds
  soaked in almond milk overnight, topped
  with sliced bananas and a sprinkle of nuts.

Lunch

- Caprese Salad with Grilled Chicken: A
  classic Caprese salad upgraded with
  grilled chicken for added protein.

Dinner

- Eggplant and Chickpea Curry: A flavorful
  vegetarian curry with eggplant, chickpeas,
  and aromatic spices.

Day 17: Nourishing & Fresh

Breakfast

- Blueberry and Almond Butter Smoothie:
  A refreshing smoothie with blueberries,
  almond butter, Greek yogurt, and a touch
  of honey.

Lunch

- Quinoa and Kale Salad with
  Lemon-Tahini Dressing: A nutrient-dense
  salad with quinoa, kale, cherry tomatoes,
  and a zesty dressing.

Dinner

- Baked Cod with Tomato and Olive Relish:
  Lightly seasoned baked cod served with a
  vibrant tomato and olive relish.

Day 18: Simple & Satisfying

Breakfast

- Peanut Butter Banana Toast: Whole-grain
  toast topped with peanut butter and sliced
  bananas.

Lunch

- Lentil and Vegetable Wrap: A fiber-rich wrap with lentils, mixed vegetables, and a drizzle of balsamic glaze.

Dinner

- Teriyaki Salmon with Broccoli and Brown Rice: Teriyaki-glazed salmon served with steamed broccoli and brown rice.

Day 19: Mediterranean Delight

Breakfast

- Mediterranean Omelette with Feta: An omelette filled with spinach, tomatoes, olives, and feta cheese.

Lunch

- Greek Chickpea Salad: A refreshing salad with chickpeas, cucumbers, cherry tomatoes, and a lemon-oregano dressing.

Dinner

- Mediterranean Stuffed Peppers: Bell
  peppers stuffed with a mixture of quinoa,
  tomatoes, olives, and herbs.

Day 20: Vibrant & Nutrient-Packed

Breakfast

- Mango and Coconut Chia Pudding: Chia
  pudding infused with mango puree and
  topped with shredded coconut.

Lunch

- Roasted Vegetable and Hummus Wrap: A
  satisfying wrap with roasted vegetables
  and a generous spread of hummus.

Dinner

- Shrimp and Quinoa Salad: A light and
  protein-packed salad with shrimp, quinoa,
  mixed greens, and a citrus vinaigrette.

Day 21: Finale of Flavor

Breakfast

- Avocado and Tomato Breakfast Sandwich: Whole-grain English muffin filled with sliced avocado, tomato, and a poached egg.

Lunch

- Spinach and Artichoke Quinoa Bowl: A flavorful bowl featuring quinoa, spinach, artichoke hearts, and a drizzle of lemon-tahini dressing.

Dinner

- Grilled Chicken Caesar Salad: Grilled chicken breast served over crisp romaine lettuce with Caesar dressing and croutons.

Week 4

Day 22: Fresh & Filling

Breakfast

- Fresh Berry Parfait: Layers of mixed berries, Greek yogurt, and granola for a delightful and nutritious breakfast.

Lunch

- Quinoa and Black Bean Salad: A protein-packed salad with quinoa, black beans, corn, tomatoes, and a lime-cilantro dressing.

Dinner

- Baked Tilapia with Lemon Herb Quinoa: Lightly seasoned tilapia baked to perfection, served with lemon herb-infused quinoa.

Day 23: Plant-Powered Goodness

Breakfast

- Green Smoothie Bowl: A nourishing bowl with a blend of spinach, banana, kiwi, and a sprinkle of seeds.

Lunch

- Chickpea and Vegetable Stir-Fry: A colorful stir-fry with chickpeas, broccoli, bell peppers, and a teriyaki glaze.

Dinner

- Stuffed Zucchini Boats: Zucchini halves filled with a mixture of ground turkey, quinoa, and diced tomatoes.

Day 24: Energizing & Satisfying

Breakfast

- Apple Cinnamon Overnight Oats: Overnight oats infused with cinnamon and topped with diced apples.

Lunch

- Mediterranean Quinoa Bowl: A Mediterranean-inspired bowl with quinoa, cherry tomatoes, cucumbers, olives, and feta cheese.

Dinner

- Lemon Garlic Shrimp with Asparagus and Brown Rice: Succulent shrimp sautéed with lemon and garlic, served with asparagus and brown rice.

Day 25: Balanced & Wholesome

Breakfast

- Almond Butter Banana Smoothie: A creamy smoothie with almond butter, banana, almond milk, and a touch of honey.

Lunch

- Lentil and Spinach Wrap: A fiber-rich wrap with lentils, spinach, tomatoes, and a drizzle of balsamic glaze.

Dinner

- Baked Chicken Breast with Quinoa and Roasted Vegetables: Simple and nutritious, baked chicken breast served with quinoa and an array of roasted vegetables.

Day 26: Fusion of Flavors

Breakfast

- Tropical Chia Seed Pudding: Chia pudding infused with tropical fruit flavors like pineapple, mango, and coconut.

Lunch

- Teriyaki Tofu and Vegetable Stir-Fry: Tofu stir-fried with a medley of colorful vegetables in a savory teriyaki sauce.

Dinner

- Cod with Tomato Basil Salsa: Baked cod topped with a refreshing tomato and basil salsa, served alongside steamed broccoli.

Day 27: Comforting & Nutrient-Rich

Breakfast

- Blueberry Banana Baked Oatmeal: Baked oatmeal filled with blueberries and banana slices.

Lunch

- Spinach and Quinoa Salad with Balsamic Glaze: A hearty salad with quinoa, baby spinach, cherry tomatoes, and a balsamic glaze.

Dinner

- Grilled Turkey Burgers with Sweet Potato Fries: Lean turkey burgers grilled to perfection, served with baked sweet potato fries.

Day 28: Finishing Strong

Breakfast

- Avocado and Berry Smoothie: A creamy smoothie with avocado, mixed berries, Greek yogurt, and a touch of honey.

Lunch

- Caprese Quinoa Salad: A quinoa salad
  with cherry tomatoes, fresh mozzarella,
  basil, and a balsamic vinaigrette.

Dinner

- Baked Salmon with Lemon Dill Sauce:
  Baked salmon fillets topped with a zesty
  lemon dill sauce, accompanied by steamed
  green beans.

Week 5

Day 29: Revitalizing Choices

Breakfast

- Kiwi and Spinach Smoothie Bowl: A
  vibrant bowl with a blend of kiwi,
  spinach, banana, and a sprinkle of seeds.

Lunch

- Chickpea and Quinoa Stuffed Bell
  Peppers: Bell peppers filled with a

flavorful mixture of chickpeas, quinoa, and Mediterranean spices.

Dinner

- Grilled Vegetable and Chickpea Salad: A light salad featuring grilled vegetables, chickpeas, and a lemon-tahini dressing.

Day 30: Savoring the Journey

Breakfast

- Mango Coconut Overnight Oats: Overnight oats infused with mango puree and coconut flakes for a tropical twist.

Lunch

- Southwest Black Bean and Corn Salad: A refreshing salad with black beans, corn, cherry tomatoes, avocado, and a lime-cilantro dressing.

Dinner

- Baked Chicken Thighs with Rosemary Roasted Potatoes: Succulent chicken thighs baked to perfection, served with rosemary-infused roasted potatoes.

Day 31: Celebratory Farewell

Breakfast

- Peanut Butter and Banana Smoothie: A satisfying smoothie with peanut butter, banana, almond milk, and a dash of cinnamon.

Lunch

- Quinoa and Chickpea Buddha Bowl: A nourishing bowl with quinoa, chickpeas, roasted vegetables, and a drizzle of tahini.

Dinner

- Grilled Swordfish with Mango Salsa: Grilled swordfish topped with a vibrant mango salsa, accompanied by a side of quinoa.

Week 6

Day 32: Refreshing Start

Breakfast

- Berry and Almond Butter Smoothie: A refreshing blend of mixed berries, almond butter, and Greek yogurt.

Lunch

- Quinoa and Avocado Salad: A hearty salad featuring quinoa, diced avocado, cherry tomatoes, and a light lemon dressing.

Dinner

- Baked Halibut with Herb-Infused Quinoa: Delicate halibut fillets baked to perfection, served alongside quinoa infused with fresh herbs.

Day 33: Energizing Boost

Breakfast

- Green Tea Infused Oatmeal: Oatmeal cooked with green tea for a unique flavor, topped with sliced kiwi and a sprinkle of chia seeds.

Lunch

- Lentil and Vegetable Stir-Fry: A colorful stir-fry with lentils, broccoli, bell peppers, and a teriyaki glaze.

Dinner

- Grilled Chicken Caesar Wrap: Grilled chicken, crisp romaine lettuce, and Caesar dressing wrapped in a whole-grain tortilla.

Day 34: Nutrient-Rich Delight

Breakfast

- Peach and Almond Smoothie Bowl: A smoothie bowl featuring fresh peaches, almond milk, and a topping of granola.

Lunch

- Mediterranean Chickpea Wrap: A satisfying wrap with chickpeas, cucumber, cherry tomatoes, and a drizzle of tzatziki sauce.

Dinner

- Baked Cod with Mango Salsa: Lightly seasoned cod baked to perfection, topped with a refreshing mango salsa.

Day 35: Wholesome & Hearty

Breakfast

- Blueberry Walnut Baked Oatmeal: Baked oatmeal with blueberries, walnuts, and a drizzle of honey.

Lunch

- Quinoa and Spinach Stuffed Bell Peppers: Bell peppers filled with a flavorful mixture of quinoa, spinach, and feta cheese.

Dinner

- Lemon Garlic Shrimp with Quinoa and Asparagus: Succulent shrimp sautéed with lemon and garlic, served with quinoa and steamed asparagus.

Day 36: Vibrant Fusion

Breakfast

- Raspberry Coconut Chia Pudding: Chia pudding infused with raspberries and coconut milk, topped with fresh raspberries.

Lunch

- Teriyaki Tofu and Vegetable Bowl: Cubes of tofu stir-fried with colorful vegetables in a teriyaki glaze, served over brown rice.

Dinner

- Baked Turkey Meatballs with Zucchini Noodles: Lean turkey meatballs baked to perfection, served over spiralized zucchini noodles.

Day 37: Comforting Choices

Breakfast

- Apple Cinnamon Whole Grain Pancakes: Fluffy pancakes made with whole grain flour, topped with sliced apples and a sprinkle of cinnamon.

Lunch

- Spinach and Chickpea Salad: A refreshing salad with baby spinach, chickpeas, cherry tomatoes, and a light balsamic vinaigrette.

Dinner

- Grilled Salmon with Lemon Dill Sauce: Grilled salmon fillets topped with a zesty lemon dill sauce, accompanied by roasted sweet potatoes.

Day 38: Nourishing & Satisfying

Breakfast

- Kiwi and Banana Smoothie: A nutrient-packed smoothie with kiwi, banana, Greek yogurt, and a touch of honey.

Lunch

- Quinoa and Black Bean Burrito Bowl: A deconstructed burrito with quinoa, black beans, corn, avocado, and salsa.

Dinner

- Baked Chicken Thighs with Quinoa and Roasted Vegetables: Tender chicken thighs baked to perfection, served with quinoa and a medley of roasted vegetables.

Day 39: Fresh & Flavorful

Breakfast

- Mango and Pineapple Overnight Oats: Overnight oats infused with tropical fruit

flavors, topped with fresh mango and
pineapple.

Lunch

- Caprese Quinoa Bowl: A quinoa bowl
  with cherry tomatoes, fresh mozzarella,
  basil, and a balsamic glaze.

Dinner

- Grilled Swordfish with Mediterranean
  Couscous: Swordfish grilled to perfection,
  served over couscous with Mediterranean
  flavors.

Day 40: Culmination of Culinary Delights

Breakfast

- Blueberry Banana Almond Butter Toast:
  Whole-grain toast topped with almond
  butter, sliced bananas, and fresh
  blueberries.

Lunch

- Greek Chickpea and Couscous Salad: A refreshing salad with chickpeas, couscous, cherry tomatoes, cucumber, and feta cheese.

Dinner

- Baked Halibut with Tomato Basil Relish: Halibut fillets baked to perfection, topped with a vibrant tomato and basil relish.

Week 7

Day 41: Savoring Simplicity

Breakfast

- Banana Nut Smoothie: A smoothie with banana, almond milk, a handful of nuts, and a dash of cinnamon.

Lunch

- Quinoa and Roasted Vegetable Wrap: A hearty wrap with quinoa, roasted vegetables, and a drizzle of balsamic glaze.

Dinner

- Teriyaki Salmon with Stir-Fried Broccoli and Brown Rice: Teriyaki-glazed salmon served with stir-fried broccoli and wholesome brown rice.

Day 42: Plant-Powered Harmony

Breakfast

- Green Goddess Avocado Toast: Whole-grain toast topped with mashed avocado, a sprinkle of seeds, and a pinch of salt.

Lunch

- Lentil and Sweet Potato Buddha Bowl: A nourishing bowl with lentils, sweet potatoes, kale, and a tahini dressing.

Dinner

- Grilled Chicken and Quinoa Salad:
  Grilled chicken breast served over a bed
  of quinoa, mixed greens, and a light
  vinaigrette.

Day 43: Fresh & Fulfilling

Breakfast

- Pineapple Coconut Chia Pudding: Chia
  pudding infused with pineapple and
  coconut milk, topped with fresh
  pineapple.

Lunch

- Mediterranean Quinoa Wrap: A flavorful
  wrap with quinoa, cherry tomatoes, olives,
  and a drizzle of tzatziki sauce.

Dinner

- Baked Cod with Lemon Garlic Asparagus:
  Lightly seasoned cod baked to perfection,
  served with lemon garlic-infused
  asparagus.

Day 44: Vibrant & Varied

Breakfast

- Mixed Berry Yogurt Parfait: Layers of mixed berries, Greek yogurt, and granola for a delightful and nutritious parfait.

Lunch

- Chickpea and Spinach Stuffed Bell Peppers: Bell peppers filled with a mixture of chickpeas, spinach, and aromatic spices.

Dinner

- Lemon Herb Grilled Shrimp with Quinoa Pilaf: Grilled shrimp marinated in lemon and herbs, served with a quinoa pilaf.

Day 45: Balanced Bliss

Breakfast

- Almond Butter and Banana Whole Grain Pancakes: Fluffy pancakes made with whole grain flour, topped with almond butter and banana slices.

Lunch

- Quinoa and Black Bean Burrito Bowl: A deconstructed burrito with quinoa, black beans, corn, avocado, and salsa.

Dinner

- Baked Chicken Thighs with Mediterranean Couscous: Tender chicken thighs baked to perfection, served over couscous with Mediterranean flavors.

Day 46: Culinary Joy

Breakfast

- Mango and Coconut Overnight Oats: Overnight oats infused with mango puree and topped with shredded coconut.

Lunch

- Greek Chickpea Salad Wrap: A refreshing wrap with chickpeas, cucumber, cherry tomatoes, and a drizzle of lemon-tahini dressing.

Dinner

- Grilled Swordfish with Tomato Basil Salsa: Swordfish grilled to perfection, topped with a vibrant tomato and basil salsa.

Day 47: Flavorful Finale

Breakfast

- Berry Medley Smoothie: A refreshing smoothie with a mix of berries, Greek yogurt, and a touch of honey.

Lunch

- Caprese Quinoa Bowl: A quinoa bowl with cherry tomatoes, fresh mozzarella, basil, and a balsamic glaze.

Dinner

- Baked Halibut with Roasted Sweet
  Potatoes: Halibut fillets baked to
  perfection, served with roasted sweet
  potatoes.

Day 48: Savoring Success

Breakfast

- Blueberry Banana Almond Butter Toast:
  Whole-grain toast topped with almond
  butter, sliced bananas, and fresh
  blueberries.

Lunch

- Greek Chickpea and Couscous Salad: A
  refreshing salad with chickpeas, couscous,
  cherry tomatoes, cucumber, and feta
  cheese.

Dinner

- Teriyaki Salmon with Quinoa and
  Steamed Broccoli: Teriyaki-glazed salmon
  served with quinoa and steamed broccoli.

Week 8

Day 49: Nutrient-Rich Fare

Breakfast

- Mixed Berry Chia Seed Smoothie: A nutrient-packed smoothie with mixed berries, chia seeds, and almond milk.

Lunch

- Quinoa and Avocado Salad: A hearty salad featuring quinoa, diced avocado, cherry tomatoes, and a light lemon dressing.

Dinner

- Baked Halibut with Herb-Infused Quinoa: Delicate halibut fillets baked to perfection, served alongside quinoa infused with fresh herbs.

Day 50: Culinary Celebration

Breakfast

- Tropical Acai Bowl: An Acai bowl infused with tropical fruits like pineapple, mango, and coconut flakes.

Lunch

- Chickpea and Quinoa Stuffed Bell Peppers: Bell peppers filled with a flavorful mixture of chickpeas, quinoa, and Mediterranean spices.

Dinner

- Grilled Vegetable and Chickpea Salad: A light salad featuring grilled vegetables, chickpeas, and a lemon-tahini dressing.

Grocery Shopping Guide

Grocery Shopping Guide

When embarking on a fertility-boosting diet, a well-planned grocery shopping list is essential to ensure you have the right ingredients on hand. Here's a comprehensive guide to help you navigate the aisles and make choices that align with your fertility goals.

1. Fresh Produce:

- Choose a variety of colorful fruits and vegetables rich in vitamins and antioxidants. Include leafy greens like spinach, kale, and Swiss chard, as well as berries, citrus fruits, avocados, and tomatoes.

2. Whole Grains:

- Opt for whole grains such as quinoa, brown rice, oats, and whole wheat products. These provide complex

carbohydrates, fiber, and essential
nutrients.

3. Lean Proteins:

- Select lean protein sources like skinless
  poultry, fish (especially those rich in
  omega-3 fatty acids like salmon), tofu,
  beans, lentils, and eggs. Protein is crucial
  for reproductive health.

4. Dairy or Dairy Alternatives:

- Include dairy products like low-fat milk,
  Greek yogurt, and cheese for calcium and
  vitamin D. Alternatively, choose fortified
  plant-based milk alternatives like almond
  or soy milk.

5. Healthy Fats:

- Incorporate sources of healthy fats such as
  avocados, nuts (almonds, walnuts), seeds
  (chia, flaxseed), and olive oil. These fats
  support hormonal balance.

6. Seafood:

- Include fatty fish like salmon, mackerel, and sardines for omega-3 fatty acids. These are beneficial for reproductive health and fetal development.

7. Beans and Legumes:

- Stock up on a variety of beans (black beans, chickpeas, lentils) and legumes. They are rich in fiber, protein, and essential nutrients.

8. Herbs and Spices:

- Enhance flavor without excess salt by using herbs (basil, cilantro, mint) and spices (turmeric, cumin, cinnamon). Herbs and spices have antioxidant properties.

9. Whole Nuts and Seeds:

- Include a mix of whole nuts (almonds, walnuts) and seeds (sunflower seeds, pumpkin seeds) for healthy snacks and additional nutrients.

10. Frozen Fruits and Vegetables:

- Keep your freezer stocked with a variety of frozen fruits and vegetables. They are convenient and retain nutritional value, offering versatility in meal preparation.

11. Whole Grain Products:

- Choose whole grain products like whole wheat bread, whole grain pasta, and brown rice. These provide a good source of fiber and essential nutrients.

12. Beverages:

- Prioritize water as your main beverage. Green tea and herbal teas are also good options. Limit sugary drinks and excessive caffeine intake.

13. Eggs:

- Eggs are a nutrient-dense source of protein and various vitamins. Include them in your diet for a well-rounded nutrition profile.

14. Prenatal Supplements:

- Consider adding prenatal supplements to your shopping list, ensuring you get essential nutrients like folic acid, iron, and vitamin D, crucial for preconception health.

15. Dairy-Free Alternatives:

- If you prefer dairy-free options, choose alternatives like almond milk, coconut milk, or soy milk. Ensure they are fortified with calcium and vitamin D.

16. Natural Sweeteners:

- Opt for natural sweeteners like honey or maple syrup in moderation. Limit the consumption of refined sugars.

17. Organic Options:

- Consider choosing organic options,
  especially for fruits and vegetables on the
  "Dirty Dozen" list to reduce exposure to
  pesticides.

18. Hydration:

- Stay well-hydrated with plenty of water.
  Consider infused water with slices of
  citrus fruits or cucumber for added flavor.

19. Miscellaneous:

- Depending on your specific meal plans,
  add any additional items like whole-grain
  flour, herbs, spices, and condiments.

Remember to check expiration dates, plan meals
in advance, and shop with a focus on fresh,
whole foods to support your fertility journey
through a nourishing and well-balanced diet.

Conclusion

Upon the conclusion of the "Fertility Diet Cookbook: Over 50 Days of Delicious Recipes to Naturally Boost Ovulation and Improve Chances of Pregnancy," I would like to sincerely thank each and every person who joined me on this culinary adventure centred on fertility. It's admirable that you decided to take an investment in your health and discover the rich world of fertility-friendly recipes. This is a positive step towards living a longer, healthier life.

We appreciate you using this cookbook as a reference. It is my genuine wish that these carefully chosen recipes have awakened your senses and given you insightful knowledge about the potent relationship between fertility and diet. Always keep in mind that cooking is a step towards improving your reproductive health and raising your chances of conceiving a healthy child.

It is encouraging to see how dedicated you are to following a diet that promotes conception. I want you to know that even though we are

finishing this book together, your opinions and
experiences count. I'm committed to carrying on
with this creative and exploratory path. In the
future, you may anticipate more recipes, tools,
and ideas on maximising your fertility and
overall wellness.
I'm wishing you luck, happiness, and prosperity
as you pursue fertility. May every dish you've
found here improve your general health and help
you achieve your most cherished goals.
With appreciation,

Steve Bell

9 798875 840517